<u>Dash diet cookbook 1:</u>

37 Meat recipes to lose weight and keep your blood pressure under control.

Christine Barberg

Meat recipes

Meat recipes

Meat recipes

Meat recipes

1) <u>Slow Cooker Barbecue Chicken Breast</u>

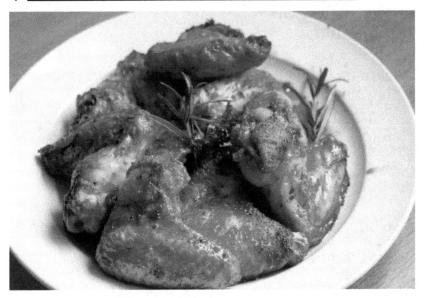

Ingredients

2 chicken breasts

1/2 teaspoon salt

1/2 teaspoon ground black pepper

1 (18 ounces) bottle barbecue sauce, divided

3 tablespoons apple cider vinegar

3 tablespoons brown sugar

1 teaspoon onion powder

1 teaspoon garlic powder

1/2 teaspoon red pepper flakes

Directions

Season chicken breasts with salt and pepper on all sides. Place in the slow cooker and pour 1/4 cup barbecue sauce and vinegar on top.

Combine brown sugar, onion powder, garlic powder, and red pepper flakes in a small bowl.

Pour out all the liquid from the slow cooker and add remaining barbecue sauce. Sprinkle chicken with brown sugar-spice mixture.

Cook on Low, occasionally stirring, until chicken is no longer pink in the center and the juices run clear about 3 more hours. An instant-read thermometer inserted into the center should read at least 165 degrees F (74 degrees C).

2) <u>Pantry Chicken Casserole</u>

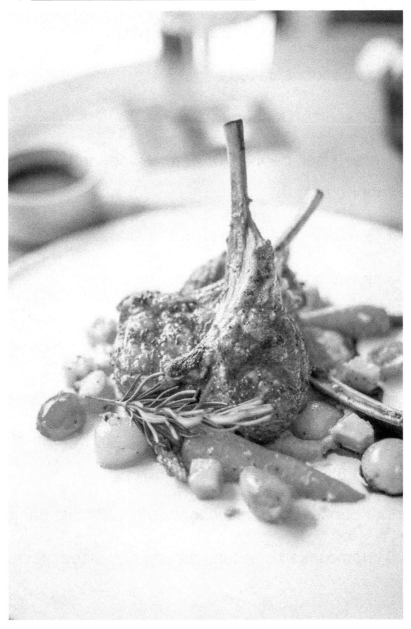

Meat recipes

Ingredients

1 (16 ounces) package penne pasta

4 tablespoons salted butter

1 large onion, chopped

1 green bell pepper - stemmed, seeded, and finely chopped

1 (8 ounces) package sliced fresh mushrooms

3 cloves garlic, minced

2 (8 ounce) packages processed cheese food (such as Velveeta®), cubed

1 (14.5 ounces) can diced tomatoes, undrained

1 (10 ounces) can dice tomatoes and green chiles (such as RO*TEL®), undrained

1 (4 ounces) can mild chopped green chile peppers

4 cups cooked chicken, cut into bite-sized pieces

Directions

Preheat the oven to 350 degrees F (175 degrees C). Spray a large casserole dish with cooking spray.

Bring a large pot of lightly salted water to a boil. Add penne and cook, occasionally stirring, until tender yet firm to the bite, about 11 minutes. Drain.

While the pasta is cooking, melt butter in a large skillet over medium heat. Add onion and bell pepper and cook, occasionally stirring, until vegetables are tender, about 5 minutes. Add mushrooms and cook until they release their liquid, about 5 minutes. Add garlic and cook, occasionally stirring, until fragrant, about 1 minute.

Stir in processed cheese food, diced tomatoes and juice, diced tomatoes and green chiles with juice, and mild chile peppers. Cook and stir until cheese has melted, 5 to 10 minutes. Remove from heat and stir in cooked pasta and chicken. Pour into the prepared baking dish.

Bake in the preheated oven until heated through, about 20 minutes. Serve warm.

3) <u>Crusted Chicken</u>

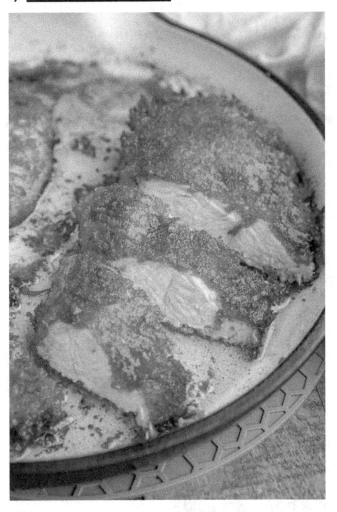

Ingredients

2 cups cheese-flavored crackers (such as Cheez-It®), crushed

1 cup French-fried onions, crushed

Meat recipes

½ cup Italian bread crumbs

2 teaspoons sesame seed, toasted

salt and ground black pepper to taste

4 skinless, boneless chicken breast halves - cut in half

3 tablespoons mayonnaise

Directions

Preheat oven to 450 degrees F (230 degrees C). Spray a baking dish with cooking spray.

Mix cheese-flavored crackers, French-fried onions, Italian bread crumbs, sesame seeds, salt, and pepper in a bowl. Set aside

Wash and pat chicken breasts dry. Spread a thin layer of mayonnaise on one side of each piece and place mayonnaise-side down in the cracker mixture.

Spread a thin layer of mayonnaise on the other side of the chicken and cover with the cracker mixture, patting firmly into the chicken. Place chicken breasts on the prepared baking dish. Sprinkle remaining cracker mixture on top; lightly spray the chicken with cooking spray.

Bake in the preheated oven until the chicken breasts are no longer pink in the center and the juices run clear 35 to 40 minutes. An instant-read thermometer inserted into the center should read at least 165 degrees F (74 degrees C).

4) <u>Slow Cooker London Broil</u>

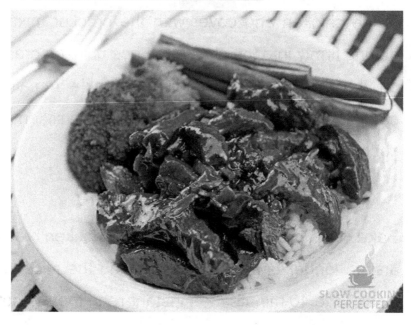

Ingredients

2 pounds flank steak

1 (10.75 ounces) can condense cream of mushroom soup

1 (10.75 ounces) can condensed tomato soup

1 (1 ounce) package dry onion soup mix

Directions

Place meat in the bottom of the slow cooker; if necessary, slice meat to make it fit!

In a medium bowl, mix together mushroom and tomato soup. Pour mixture over beef. Sprinkle dry onion soup mix over the top.

5) <u>Korean Barbecued Short Ribs:</u>

Crosscut beef short ribs, don't hesitate to substitute another cut of beef, for example, sirloin or toss, cut 1/4-inch thick across the grain. The marinade is likewise great on rib-eyes, skirt steak, and even chicken thighs or bosoms.

Ingredients:

1) 1/2 Cup soy sauce

2) 1/2 Cup water

3) 2 tablespoons white vinegar or rice vinegar

4) 2 tablespoons earthy colored sugar

5) 1 tablespoon granulated sugar or honey

6) 2 Cloves garlic, minced

7) 1 ready pear, stripped, cored, and coarsely hacked

8) 1 1-INCh piece new ginger, stripped and cut into coins

9) 1 Scallion (green onion), managed and coarsely slashed

10)   2 teaspoons sesame oil

11)   1 teaspoon Traeger Beef Shake, or salt

Method:

1) Lay the beef in a solitary layer in a heating dish and season on both sides with Traeger Beef Shake. Pour the marinade over the beef, surrendering the beef to cover the two sides. Cover and refrigerate for a few hours, or

overnight.

2) When prepared to cook, start the Traeger barbecue on Smoke with the cover open until the fire is set up.

3) Remove the beef from the marinade; dispose of marinade. Mastermind the beef on the flame broil mesh and barbecue, 2 to 3 minutes for every side, or until the meat is cooked however you would prefer. (In Korea, they favor their short ribs very much done.)

6) Italian Meatball Subs:

These sandwiches are for good cravings—ideal for game day or a bustling weeknight dinner. You can likewise shape the meat combination into mixed drink size meatballs (utilize smaller than expected biscuit tins to heat them for roughly 20 minutes) and serve on toothpicks with warm marinara as a plunging sauce.

Ingredients:

1) 1-1/2 pounds ground beef
2) ½ pound-mass Italian hotdog or ground pork
3) 3/4 cup prepared dry bread scraps
4) 1/2 cup ground Parmesan
5) 1/4 cup onion, finely minced
6) 2 cloves garlic, finely minced
7) 1 egg, daintily
8) Your most loved jolted spaghetti or marinara sauce
9) 4 hoagie or sub moves split through the side

Meat recipes

7) <u>Meat and vegetables</u>

Serves 2

Ingredients:

1) 1/2 cup earthy colored rice
2) 2 cups water
3) 4 ounces top sirloin (decision)
4) 3 tablespoons without fat Italian dressing
5) 1 green pepper, cultivated and cut into 4 pieces
6) 4 cherry tomatoes
7) 1 little onion, cut into 4 wedges
8) 2 wooden sticks, absorbed water for 30 minutes, or metal sticks

Method:

1) In a pot over high warmth, consolidate the rice and water. Heat to the point of boiling. Lessen the warmth to low, cover, and stew until the water is ingested and the rice is delicate

around 30 to 45 minutes. Add more water if important to shield the rice from drying out. Move to a little bowl to keep warm.

2) Cut the meat into 4 equivalent parts. Put the meat in a little dumbfound and pour Italian dressing on the top. Put in the fridge for in any event 20 minutes to marinate, turning to vary.

3) Set up a fire in a charcoal barbecue or warmth a gas flame broil or an oven. Away from the warmth source, delicately cover the barbecue rack or grill skillet with a cooking shower. Position the cooking rack 4 to 6 creeps from the warmth source.

4) String 2 blocks of meat, 2 green pepper cuts, 2 cherry tomatoes, and 2 onion wedges onto each stick. Spot the kebabs on the barbecue rack or grill container. Barbecue or sear the kebabs for around 5 to 10 minutes, turning to

vary.

8) <u>Sauteed Scallops</u>

Ingredients:

1) 1 lb frozen sound scallops, defrosted, washed and wipe off 1 tsp parsley, hacked
2) 1 tsp lemon juice
3) 1 tsp garlic, minced
4) 2 tbsp olive oil
5) Pepper
6) Salt

Method:

1) Warm oil in a dish over medium warmth.

2) Add garlic and sauté for 30 seconds.

3) Add scallops, lemon squeeze, pepper, and

salt, and sauté until scallops turn dark. Trimming with parsley and serve.

9) Bacon-Wrapped Egg Cups

To give this recipe a little kick, replace the Cheddar cheese with pepper jack and add a pinch of red pepper flakes to the eggs while you're whisking.

PER SERVING Calories: 187 | Fat: 13.1g | Protein: 12.5g | Sodium: 398mg | Fiber: 0.9g | Carbohydrates: 2.6g | Sugar: 0.9g

INGREDIENTS | SERVES 12

12 slices sugar-free bacon

12 large eggs

1/2 cup heavy cream

1/2 teaspoon salt

1/4 teaspoon black pepper

1/2 cup shredded Cheddar cheese

2 cups chopped and steamed broccoli

1. Preheat oven to 350°F.

2. Grease each well of a 12-cup muffin tin with butter or coconut oil.

3. Cook bacon in a medium skillet over medium heat until almost crisp. When bacon is fully cooked, quickly line each well of the muffin tin with a piece of bacon.

4. Whisk eggs, heavy cream, salt, and pepper together in a large mixing bowl. Add cheese and chopped broccoli and stir.

5. Pour an equal amount of mixture into each well of the muffin tin.

6. Bake for 20 minutes or until lightly browned on top and firm throughout.

7. Allow to cool for 10 minutes and then remove egg cups from muffin tins. Store in refrigerator.

Be Choosy with Bacon

Like commercially prepared sausage, bacon often contains added sugar in the form of maple syrup or brown sugar. Look for uncured varieties at the supermarket or ask your local butcher to track down some sugar-free bacon for you.

10)   Bacon Hash

Turn this into a complete meal by adding a couple of poached or over-easy eggs on top. You can also mix this bacon hash into some scrambled eggs.

PER SERVING Calories: 107 | Fat: 5.9g | Protein: 7.3g | Sodium: 597mg | Fiber: 1.6g | Carbohydrates: 6.2g | Sugar: 2.1g

INGREDIENTS | SERVES 4

6 slices sugar-free bacon

2 cups chopped cauliflower

1 medium onion, diced

2 cloves garlic, minced

1/2 teaspoon salt

1/2 teaspoon black pepper

1/2 teaspoon garlic powder

1. Cook bacon in a medium skillet over medium heat until crispy, about 10 minutes. Remove from pan and let cool, then dice.

2. Add cauliflower, onion, and garlic to the skillet. Cook 5 minutes over medium heat, or until cauliflower starts to brown. Add salt, black pepper, garlic powder, and diced bacon. Stir until combined.

3. Remove from heat and serve.

11) Scrambled Eggs

This is a simple recipe, but it's a staple for a ketogenic diet. Scrambled eggs and bacon are typically thought of as breakfast food, but you can eat this whenever you need a quick dose of protein and fat.

PER SERVING Calories: 425 | Fat: 31.2g | Protein: 27.3g | Sodium: 901mg | Fiber: 0.1g | Carbohydrates: 2.5g | Sugar: 1.4g

INGREDIENTS | SERVES 2

4 slices sugar-free bacon

6 large eggs

1/4 cup heavy cream

1/4 teaspoon salt

1/4 teaspoon black pepper

1. Cook bacon in a medium skillet over medium heat until crispy, about 10 minutes. Remove bacon from pan and dice.

2. Crack eggs into a medium bowl and whisk together with heavy cream, salt, and pepper. Add egg mixture to bacon grease in pan and stir until scrambled. Add diced bacon to eggs and stir.

3. Remove from heat and serve immediately.

12)   Sausage Quiche

This quiche holds up well in the fridge, so it's a good choice when meal planning. You can prepare the quiche on Sunday, put each serving in a plastic container in the fridge, and eat it for breakfast all week.

PER SERVING Calories: 262 | Fat: 18.9g | Protein: 16.3g | Sodium: 633mg | Fiber: 0.0g | Carbohydrates: 2.0g | Sugar: 0.6g

INGREDIENTS | SERVES 12

12 large eggs

1/4 cup heavy cream

1/2 teaspoon salt

1/4 teaspoon black pepper

12 ounces sugar-free breakfast sausage

2 cups shredded Cheddar cheese

1. Preheat oven to 375°F.

2. Whisk eggs, heavy cream, salt, and pepper together in a large bowl.

3. Add breakfast sausage and Cheddar cheese.

4. Pour mixture into a greased 9" × 13" casserole dish.

5. Bake for 25 minutes. Cut into 12 squares and serve.

13)   Ham, Cheese, and Egg Casserole

Mozzarella and Cheddar cheese give this dish a mild cheesy flavor, but you can use any type of shredded cheese you want.

PER SERVING Calories: 296 | Fat: 15.8g | Protein: 30.1g | Sodium: 893mg | Fiber: 0.1g | Carbohydrates: 3.8g | Sugar: 0.6g

INGREDIENTS | SERVES 6

4 cups broccoli florets

12 large eggs

2 cups cooked diced sugar-free ham

1/2 cup shredded mozzarella cheese

1/2 cup shredded Cheddar cheese

1/4 cup chopped scallions

1. Preheat oven to 375°F.

2. Fill a large pot with water and bring to a boil. Blanch broccoli by putting in boiling water for 2–3 minutes.

3. Put eggs, ham, mozzarella, Cheddar, and scallions in a large bowl and whisk until combined. Add broccoli.

4. Pour into a 9" × 13" baking dish and cook for 35 minutes or until eggs are cooked through.

14)   <u>Bacon-and-Egg-Stuffed Avocados</u>

Take these stuffed avocados out of the oven as soon as the egg is cooked through. If you cook an avocado too long, it develops a bitter, unpleasant taste.

PER SERVING Calories: 478 | Fat: 35.1g | Protein: 23.1g | Sodium: 830mg | Fiber: 9.3g | Carbohydrates: 13.1g | Sugar: 0.8g

INGREDIENTS | SERVES 2

2 large avocados

4 strips cooked sugar-free bacon, crumbled

4 large eggs

1/4 teaspoon sea salt

1/4 teaspoon black pepper

1. Preheat oven to 400°F.

2. Cut avocados in half lengthwise and remove the pit. Scoop some avocado out of each half to create a well.

3. Sprinkle 1 strip crumbled bacon into each avocado well. Crack 1 egg directly into each avocado half. Season with salt and black pepper. Place avocados on a baking sheet.

4. Bake for 15 minutes or until egg is cooked to desired doneness.

A for Avocado

Avocados are the ketogenic dieter's dream. A single avocado contains almost 30 grams of fat and only 3 grams of net carbohydrates. You can easily increase the fat content of any meal by adding a few slices of avocado.

15) <u>Mediterranean Rollups</u>

Olives and sun-dried tomatoes are the flavors of the Mediterranean Sea. From Italy to Greece, the tastes of hot summer days include ripe tomatoes and fresh olive oil, and the scent of beautiful olive groves. This recipe will take you there!

PER 1 FAT BOMB Calories: 155 | Fat: 12.6g | Protein: 3.9g | Sodium: 502mg | Fiber: 1.9g | Carbohydrates: 4.9g | Sugar: 0.1g

INGREDIENTS | MAKES 2 FAT BOMBS

1 large egg

1 tablespoon extra-virgin olive oil

1/8 teaspoon sea salt

6 large kalamata olives, pitted

1 ounce sun-dried tomatoes in oil

1/8 teaspoon red chili flakes

1/8 teaspoon parsley flakes

Meat recipes

1. In a small bowl, combine egg, olive oil, and salt and whisk until foamy.

2. Heat a small nonstick skillet over high heat and pour in egg mixture, spreading evenly so it forms a thin, even layer.

3. Once the first side is cooked, about 1 minute, flip frittata with the aid of a plate or a lid. Cook until golden on bottom, about 2 more minutes.

4. Remove frittata to a plate.

5. In a small food processor, mix olives, tomatoes, chili flakes, and parsley flakes until well chopped and blended, about 30 seconds.

6. Spread olive paste on top of frittata in an even layer.

7. Roll frittata into a tight roll, cut into 2 pieces, and serve immediately

16)   Egg, Sausage, and Chorizo Bacon Cups

These classic flavors combine to make a portable, low-carbohydrate breakfast bowl. This bowl is a truly filling meal for any pork lover on the run.

PER 1 FAT BOMB Calories: 258 | Fat: 18.6g | Protein: 16.7g | Sodium: 901mg | Fiber: 0.1g | Carbohydrates: 1.4g | Sugar: 0.5g

INGREDIENTS | MAKES 6 FAT BOMBS

12 slices regular-cut bacon, 6 cut in half

4 large eggs

1/2 teaspoon salt

2 tablespoons freshly chopped cilantro

4 ounces raw breakfast sausage

2 ounces chorizo, diced

1/4 small yellow onion, peeled and diced

Meat recipes

1. Preheat oven to 400°F.

2. In a standard-sized muffin tin, place half-strips bacon in an X shape in the bottom of 6 cups.

3. Line those same cups with a full slice of bacon along the inside of the cup vertically.

4. Place a cookie sheet underneath muffin tin and bake cups 8–10 minutes until they're a little pliable.

5. While cups are precooking, whisk eggs with salt and cilantro in a medium bowl. Set aside.

6. Combine breakfast sausage, chorizo, and onions in small mixing bowl.

7. Take cups out of oven and divide chorizo and sausage mixture equally between cups.

8. Pour egg mixture over sausage mixture and return cups to oven.

9. Bake cups 12–15 minutes more until eggs set. Serve warm.

17) <u>Egg, Sour Cream, and Chive Bacon Cups</u>

Sour cream is an excellent way to add extra fat to your fat bombs, and to make scrambled eggs taste even creamier. Chives enhance the flavor to make this cup even better than a potato chip with a similar name.

PER 1 FAT BOMB Calories: 163 | Fat: 11.3g | Protein: 12.1g | Sodium: 533mg | Fiber: 0.5g | Carbohydrates: 0.9g | Sugar: 0.3g

INGREDIENTS | MAKES 6 FAT BOMBS

12 slices regular-cut bacon, 6 cut in half

4 large eggs

1/2 teaspoon salt

1/4 teaspoon freshly ground black pepper

2 tablespoons diced chives

2 tablespoons sour cream

Meat recipes

1. Preheat oven to 400°F.

2. In a standard-sized muffin tin, place half-strips in an X shape in the bottom of 6 cups. Line those same cups with 1 full slice bacon along the inside of the cup vertically.

3. Place a cookie sheet underneath muffin tin and bake cups 8–10 minutes until they're a little pliable.

4. While cups are precooking, whisk eggs with remaining ingredients in a medium bowl. Set aside.

5. Take cups out of oven and divide egg mixture equally between cups.

6. Bake cups 8–10 minutes more until eggs set. Serve warm.

18)   Ham and Cheese Casserole

Allow the cream cheese to reach room temperature before starting this recipe. Softened cream cheese is much easier to work with than cream cheese fresh from the fridge.

PER SERVING Calories: 355 | Fat: 23.6g | Protein: 23.2g | Sodium: 1,223mg | Fiber: 2.3g | Carbohydrates: 7.8g | Sugar: 3.7g

INGREDIENTS | SERVES 6

6 cups cauliflower florets

1/2 cup cream cheese, softened

1/2 cup heavy cream

1/4 cup coconut cream

21/2 cups cooked cubed sugar-free ham

1 cup shredded Cheddar cheese

11/2 tablespoons grated Parmesan cheese

1/4 cup chopped scallions

1/2 teaspoon salt

1/4 teaspoon black pepper

Meat recipes

1. Preheat oven to 350°F. Bring a large pot of water to a boil and add cauliflower. Boil until cauliflower is fork tender, about 5–10 minutes. Strain cauliflower and return to pot.

2. Put cream cheese, heavy cream, and coconut cream in a medium mixing bowl and beat with a handheld beater until smooth. Transfer cream cheese mixture to cauliflower pot and stir until cauliflower is coated. Add in ham, Cheddar cheese, Parmesan cheese, scallions, salt, and pepper and stir until combined.

3. Transfer mixture to a 9" × 9" baking dish and bake until cheese is melted and casserole is bubbly, about 30 minutes. Serve hot.

19)   <u>Spicy Chicken and Avocado Casserole</u>

You can replace the chicken in this recipe with canned tuna, ground beef or pork, or diced chunks of ham.

PER SERVING Calories: 533 | Fat: 40.1g | Protein: 29.0g | Sodium: 1,031mg | Fiber: 3.5g | Carbohydrates: 6.7g | Sugar: 1.6g

INGREDIENTS | SERVES 6

2 large avocados, roughly chopped

2 tablespoons coconut oil

1 small onion, diced

1 medium green bell pepper, diced

3 (12.5-ounce) cans shredded chicken breast

1/2 cup sour cream

1/2 cup Homemade Mayonnaise (see recipe in Chapter 5)

11/2 cups shredded Cheddar cheese, divided

1/8 teaspoon red pepper flakes

1/4 teaspoon salt

1/4 teaspoon black pepper

1. Preheat oven to 350°F.

2. Spread chopped avocados along the bottom of a 9" × 13" baking pan.

3. Heat coconut oil in a medium skillet over medium-high heat. Add onions and cook until lightly browned, about 3 minutes. Add bell pepper to pan and cook until soft, another 3 minutes. Remove from heat.

4. Place chicken, sour cream, mayonnaise, 1 cup of Cheddar cheese, red pepper flakes, salt, and black pepper in a medium mixing bowl and stir until combined. Add onions and bell peppers.

5. Spoon mixture over avocados. Top with remaining 1/2 cup of Cheddar cheese.

6. Bake for 20 minutes, or until cheese is slightly browned and casserole is bubbling.

7. Allow to cool slightly before serving.

Go Crazy for Coconut Oil

Coconut oil is a staple in the ketogenic diet. The oil is resistant to high heat, so unlike olive oil, it doesn't oxidize with high temperatures. Coconut oil also contains medium-chain triglycerides, a type of fat that can help boost metabolism.

DIRECTIONS :

1.Preheat the waffle maker.

2.Add the eggs, cream cheese, mozzarella cheese, salt and pepper, dried dill, onion powder and garlic powder to a bowl.

3.Mix everything with a fork just until batter forms.

4.Rub butter onthe heated waffle maker and add a few tablespoons of the batter.

5.Cover and cook for about 7 minutes depending on your waffle maker.

6.Meanwhile, heat some butter in a nonstick pan.

7.Season the chicken with salt and pepper and sprinkle with dried dill. Pour the heavy cream on top.

8.Cook the chicken slices for about 10 minutes or until golden brown.

9.Cut each chaffle in half.

10.On one half add a lettuce leaf, tomato slice, and chicken slice. Cover with the other chaffle half to make a sandwich.

11.Serve and enjoy.

NUTRITION:

Calories 537, fat 37.3 g, carbs 5.5 g, sugar 0.6 g,Protein 44.3 g, sodium 328 m g

20) <u>Creamy Bacon Salad on A Chaffle:</u>

Preparation time : 10 minutes

Cooking Time :15 Minutes

Servings : 2

INGREDIENTS :

4 eggs

1½ cups grated mozzarella cheese

½ cup parmesan cheese

Salt and pepper to taste

1 teaspoon dried oregano

¼ cup almond flour

2 teaspoons baking powder

Bacon salad

½ pound cooked bacon

1 cup cream cheese

1 teaspoon dried oregano

1 teaspoon dried basil

1 teaspoon dried rosemary

2 tablespoons lemon juice

2 tablespoons butter

2 spring onions, finely chopped, for serving

DIRECTIONS :

1. Preheat the waffle maker.

2. Add the eggs, mozzarella cheese, parmesan cheese, salt and pepper, dried oregano, almond flour and baking powder to a bowl.

3. Mix thoroughly.

4. Rub butter on the heated waffle maker and add a few tablespoons of the batter.

5. Cover and cook for about 7 minutes depending on your waffle maker.

6. Meanwhile, chop the cooked bacon into smaller pieces and place them in a bowl with the cream cheese. Season with dried oregano, dried basil, dried rosemary and lemon juice.

7. Mix until combined and spread each chaffle with the creamy bacon salad.

8.To serve, sprinkle some freshly chopped spring onion on top.

NUTRITION:

Calories 750, fat 62.5 g, carbs 7.7 g, sugar 0.8 g, Protein 40.3 g, sodium 1785 mg

21) <u>Beef and Sour Cream :</u>

Preparation time : 10 minutes

Cooking Time :15 Minutes

Servings : 2

INGREDIENTS :

Butter

4 eggs

2 cups grated mozzarella cheese

3 tablespoons coconut flour

3 tablespoons almond flour

2 teaspoons baking powder

Salt and pepper to taste

1 tablespoon freshly chopped parsley

Seasoned beef

1 pound beef tenderloin

Salt and pepper to taste

2 tablespoons olive oil

1 tablespoon Dijon mustard

Other

2 tablespoons olive oil to brush the waffle maker

¼ cup sour cream for garnish

2 tablespoons freshly chopped spring onion for garnish

DIRECTIONS :

2.Add the eggs, grated mozzarella cheese, coconut flour, almond flour, baking powder, salt and pepper and freshly chopped parsley to a bowl.

3.Mix until just combined and batter forms.

5.Cover and cook for about 7 minutes depending on your waffle maker.

6.Meanwhile, heat the olive oil in a nonstick pan over medium heat.

7.Season the beef tenderloin with salt and pepper and spread the whole piece of beef tenderloin with Dijon mustard.

10.Garnish with freshly chopped spring onion.11.Serve and enjoy.

NUTRITION:

Calories 543, fat 37 g, carbs 7.9 g, sugar 0.5 g,Protein 44.9 g, sodium 269 m g

22)   <u>Beef Sandwich Recipe:</u>

Preparation time : 10 minutes

Cooking Time :15 Minutes

Servings : 2

INGREDIENTS :

Butter

3 eggs

2 cups grated mozzarella cheese

¼ cup cream cheese

Salt and pepper to taste

1 teaspoon Italian seasoning

Beef

2 tablespoons butter

1 pound beef tenderloin

Salt and pepper to taste

2 teaspoons Dijon mustard

1 teaspoon dried paprika

Other

2 tablespoons cooking spray to brush the waffle maker

4 lettuce leaves for serving

4 tomato slices for serving

4 leaves fresh basil

DIRECTIONS :

2.Add the eggs, grated mozzarella cheese, salt and pepper and Italian seasoning to a bowl.

3.Mix until combined and butter forms.

5.Cover and cook for about 7 minutes depending on your waffle maker.

6.Meanwhile, melt and heat the butter in a nonstick frying pan.

7.Season the beef loin with salt and pepper, brush it with Dijon mustard, and sprinkle some dried paprika on top.

8.Cook the beef on each side for about 5 minutes.

9.Thinly slice the beef and assemble the sandwiches.

NUTRITION:

Calories 477, fat 32.8g, carbs 2.3 g, sugar 0.9 g, Protein 42.2 g, sodium 299 m g

23)   <u>Turkey Avocado Rolls</u>

Lemon pepper has a strong taste, so in this recipe, a little goes a long way. If you don't like the zing of lemon, try garlic pepper in place of the lemon pepper or just omit the spice blend completely.

PER SERVING Calories: 689 | Fat: 49.3g | Protein: 47.6g | Sodium: 424mg | Fiber: 2.8g | Carbohydrates: 8.6g | Sugar: 1.4g

INGREDIENTS | SERVES 4

12 (1-ounce) slices turkey breast

12 slices Swiss cheese

3 cups baby spinach

1 large avocado, cut into 12 slices

1/4 cup Homemade Mayonnaise (see recipe in Chapter 5)

1/4 teaspoon lemon pepper

Meat recipes

1. Lay out the slices of turkey breast flat and place a slice of Swiss cheese on top of each one.

2. Top each slice with 1/4 cup baby spinach and 1 slice of avocado. Drizzle with 1 teaspoon of mayonnaise.

3. Sprinkle each "sandwich" with lemon pepper. Roll up sandwiches and secure with toothpicks. Serve immediately or refrigerate until ready to serve.

Check Your Spices

It may come as a surprise, but many commercial spices contain sugar or hydrogenated fats. Don't assume that an ingredient, such as lemon pepper, is free of carbohydrates until you check the label. If it contains sugar, ditch it and find one that doesn't. When it comes to herbs and spices, there are plenty of sugar-free options out there.

24)   <u>Chicken Casserole</u>

Traditional chicken cordon bleu contains ham, chicken, and Swiss cheese, but if you're not a fan of Swiss cheese, swap it out for a cheese with a milder flavor, such as provolone or mozzarella.

PER SERVING Calories: 584 | Fat: 38.9g | Protein: 44.0g | Sodium: 927mg | Fiber: 0.1g | Carbohydrates: 5.2g | Sugar: 3.1g

INGREDIENTS | SERVES 4

2 cups cooked chopped chicken breast

1 cup cooked diced sugar-free ham

1 cup cubed Swiss cheese

1/2 cup heavy cream

1/2 cup sour cream

1/2 cup cream cheese

1/2 teaspoon granulated garlic

1/2 teaspoon granulated onion

1/4 teaspoon salt

1/4 teaspoon black pepper

1 ounce crushed pork rinds

1. Preheat oven to 350°F.

2. Mix chicken and ham and spread out in the bottom of a 9" × 13" baking dish.

3. Sprinkle Swiss cheese on top of chicken and ham.

4. Put heavy cream, sour cream, and cream cheese in a medium saucepan and heat over medium heat until cream cheese is melted and mixture is smooth. Add garlic, onion, salt, and pepper. Pour mixture over chicken, ham, and Swiss cheese.

5. Sprinkle pork rinds across casserole. Bake for 30 minutes, or until slightly browned and cheese is bubbly.

25)   <u>Stuffed Chicken Breast</u>

You can use frozen spinach in place of the fresh spinach for this recipe. Just make sure it's completely thawed and drained before use or the filling will be runny.

PER SERVING Calories: 271 | Fat: 12.7g | Protein: 30.8g | Sodium: 346mg | Fiber: 1.7g | Carbohydrates: 4.7g | Sugar: 1.3g

INGREDIENTS | SERVES 4

1 pound (4 individual) boneless, skinless chicken breasts

1/4 cup cream cheese, softened

1/4 cup sour cream

1 (10-ounce) package fresh spinach, chopped

1/3 cup chopped fresh basil

1 tablespoon minced green onions

1/2 cup shredded pepper jack cheese

Meat recipes

2 cloves garlic, minced

1/4 teaspoon salt

1/4 teaspoon black pepper

1. Preheat oven to 375°F.

2. Cut a slit into the side of each chicken breast to create a pocket.

3. Combine all other ingredients in a medium bowl and beat until smooth.

4. Fill each chicken breast with 1/4 of the mixture and secure pocket closed with toothpicks.

5. Place chicken breasts in a baking dish and cook for 35 minutes, or until chicken is no longer pink.

26) <u>Meatloaf</u>

You don't need bread crumbs to hold meatloaf together. This recipe uses an egg instead, which keeps the carbohydrates low while also increasing fat and protein content.

PER SERVING Calories: 321 | Fat: 19.5g | Protein: 25.7g | Sodium: 566mg | Fiber: 0.8g | Carbohydrates: 4.7g | Sugar: 1.5g

INGREDIENTS | SERVES 4

2 tablespoons butter

1 large yellow onion

4 cloves garlic, minced

4 slices cooked sugar-free bacon

1 pound 85/15 lean ground beef

1 large egg

1 teaspoon dried thyme

1 teaspoon dried parsley

1/2 teaspoon dry mustard

1/2 teaspoon salt

1/4 teaspoon black pepper

1. Preheat oven to 350°F.

2. Heat butter in a large skillet over medium-high heat until melted. Add onions and garlic and sauté until softened, 3–4 minutes. Remove from heat and set aside to cool.

3. Chop bacon and put in a large mixing bowl. Add ground beef, egg, herbs, spices, and garlic and onion mixture and mix until evenly incorporated.

4. Transfer meat mixture to a 9" × 5" loaf pan.

5. Cook for 1 hour or until a meat thermometer inserted in the center reads 165°F.

Parsley isn't just a garnish. The herb is rich in vitamin C and vitamin A, so it helps keep your immune system, bones, and nervous system strong. Parsley also helps flush out excess water from the body and keeps your kidneys healthy.

27)   <u>Burger Chaffle:</u>

Preparation time : 5 minutes

Cooking Time : 10 Minutes

Servings : 2

INGREDIENTS :

1/3 lb beef, ground

½ tsp garlic salt

3 slices of cheese you prefer

Salt and ground pepper to taste

Assembling:

2 tbsp lettuce, shredded

4 dill pickles

2 tsp onion, minced

DIRECTIONS :

1.Take your burger patties. Top with shredded lettuce, onions and pickles.

2.Spread the sauce over and place it on top of the veggies, sauce side down.

3.Enjoy.

NUTRITION:

Calories per Servings : 850 Kcal ; Fats: 56 g ; Carbs: 8 g ; Protein: 67 g

28)   <u>Beef Bowls</u>

If you prefer to mimic more traditional tacos, you can place the filling for this recipe into large leaves of iceberg lettuce and fold them up like tacos.

PER SERVING Calories: 494 | Fat: 33.7g | Protein: 28.5g | Sodium: 704mg | Fiber: 3.4g | Carbohydrates: 8.5g | Sugar: 2.3g

INGREDIENTS | SERVES 4

1 pound 85/15 lean ground beef

2 tablespoons taco seasoning

1 large avocado, chopped

1 cup shredded Cheddar cheese

1 cup sour cream

1/2 cup sliced black olives

Cilantro, chopped (optional)

1. Brown ground beef in a large skillet over medium heat. Without draining fat, add taco seasoning and stir until liquid is absorbed and beef is covered with seasoning.

2. Put 1/4 of the beef into each of four bowls. Top beef in each bowl with 1/4 avocado, 1/4 cup of Cheddar cheese, 1/4 cup of sour cream, and 1/8 cup of sliced olives.

3. Garnish with cilantro, if desired.

Whenever possible, choose high-quality meats such as grass-fed beef and free-range, organic chicken. Animals that consume their natural diet are better for you nutritionally.

29) <u>Garlic Roasted Chicken and Potatoes</u>

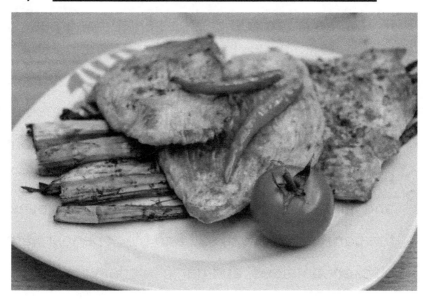

Ingredients

¼ cup butter

6 chicken leg quarters, split into drumsticks and thighs

6 large Yukon Gold potatoes, cut into chunks

24 cloves garlic, unpeeled

1 pinch salt and ground black pepper to taste

¼ cup maple syrup

Directions

Preheat oven to 400 degrees F (200 degrees C).

Place the butter into a roasting pan, and melt in the oven. When butter is melted, swirl to coat the bottom of the roasting pan and place the chicken drumsticks and thighs, potatoes, and unpeeled garlic cloves into the pan. Sprinkle with salt and black pepper; turn the chicken, potatoes, and garlic to coat with butter.

Bake in the preheated oven until the chicken is no longer pink inside and the juices run clear, about 40 minutes, basting 3 times with pan drippings. Brush maple syrup over the chicken pieces, and spoon pan drippings over the potatoes.

Return to oven and bake until the chicken and potatoes are tender and browned about 20 more minutes. An instant-read thermometer inserted into a thick part of a thigh should read at least 165 degrees F (74 degrees C). To serve, squeeze garlic from the baked cloves and spread the soft garlic over the chicken. Pour pan juices over chicken and potatoes.

30)   <u>**French Sandwiches (Slow Cooker)**</u>

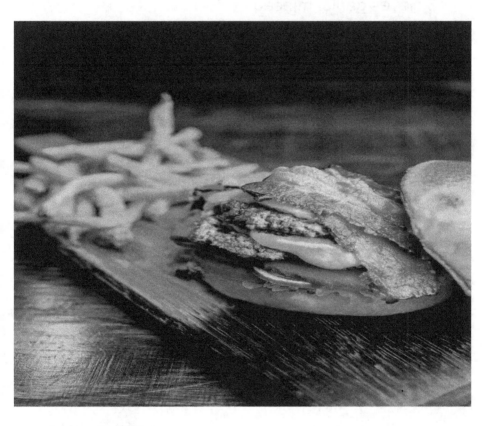

Ingredients

5 tablespoons olive oil, divided

Meat recipes

2 large onions, thinly sliced

3 tablespoons butter, divided

1 teaspoon white sugar

½ teaspoon salt

3 cloves garlic, minced

9 tablespoons water

¼ cup dry vermouth

2 ½ cups beef stock

1 tablespoon Worcestershire sauce

1 tablespoon soy sauce

1 teaspoon fresh thyme

1 bay leaf

¼ teaspoon ground black pepper

3 pounds rump roast

salt and ground black pepper to taste

8 French rolls, split

1 (6 ounces) package grated Gruyere cheese

Directions

Heat 3 tablespoons olive oil over medium heat in a large, deep pot. Add onions and toss to coat with oil. Cook, often stirring, until softened, about 15 minutes. Add 1 tablespoon butter. Cook and stir until onions start to brown, about 15 minutes more.

Stir sugar and 1/2 teaspoon salt into the onions in the pot. Continue to cook, stirring once halfway through, until onions are well-browned, 10 to 15 minutes more. Mix in garlic and cook for 1 minute more.

Stir 3 tablespoons of water into the pot, scraping bits from the bottom. Let simmer for 3 minutes; repeat with an additional 3 tablespoons water. Simmer for 3 minutes more and repeat. Add vermouth; scrape bits from the bottom and sides of the pot. Cook for 4 minutes more. Add stock, Worcestershire sauce, soy sauce, thyme, and bay leaf. Simmer for 10 minutes; do not boil. Add black pepper. Discard bay leaf. Remove pot from heat and allow soup to cool. Pour into the slow cooker, but don't turn it on.

Trim any excess fat from the rump roast. Sprinkle all sides with salt and pepper—heat remaining 2 tablespoons olive oil in the pot over high heat. Cook the meat, holding it down with tongs until browned on all sides, about 10 minutes. Transfer meat carefully to the slow cooker. Spoon the soup over the meat so that it is topped with a few onions. Cover and cook on Low for 4 hours.

Remove meat from the slow cooker. Slice it diagonally and return slices to the slow cooker. Continue to cook on Low for 2 hours more.

Meat recipes

Preheat the oven to 350 degrees F (175 degrees C). Spread rolls with remaining 2 tablespoons butter; place face-down on a baking sheet.

Bake rolls in the preheated oven until beginning to brown, 8 to 10 minutes. Remove from the oven, flip, and sprinkle with Gruyere cheese. Set an oven rack about 6 inches from the heat source and turn on the oven's broiler. Broil rolls until cheese is slightly bubbly and lightly browned 2 to 4 minutes.

Remove meat from the slow cooker using a slotted spoon. Place on the rolls. Serve soup on the side for dipping.

31)   <u>Chicken Salad</u>

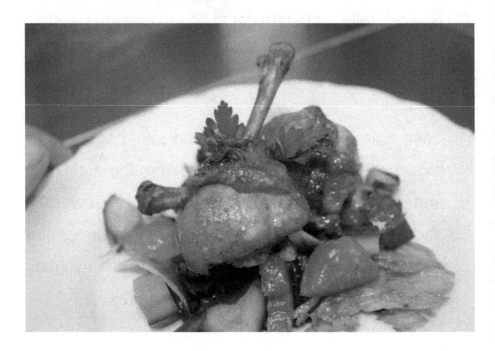

Ingredients

1 (6 ounces) package smoked chicken breast, skin removed, cubed

1 cup seedless grapes, halved

½ cup diced red onion

3 stalks celery, diced

¼ cup fresh basil leaves, cut into thin strips

1 cup blanched slivered almonds

¾ cup mayonnaise

Directions

In a large bowl, combine the smoked chicken, grapes, red onion, celery, basil, almonds, and mayonnaise. Mix well; chill and serve.

32) <u>Mushroom-Stuffed Chicken Breasts</u>

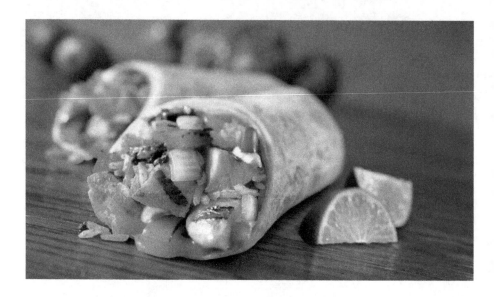

Ingredients

4 eaches skinless, boneless chicken breast halves

2 tablespoons butter

1 (8 ounces) package baby portabella mushrooms, sliced

2 cloves garlic, minced

½ teaspoon thyme

1 (8 ounces) package cream cheese

¼ teaspoon salt

toothpicks

2 tablespoons Dijon mustard

2 tablespoons grated Parmesan cheese, or as needed

Directions

Preheat the oven to 400 degrees F (200 degrees C). Set an oven rack in the center of the oven.

Place chicken breasts between 2 sheets of heavy plastic on a solid, level surface. Firmly pound with the smooth side of a meat mallet to 1/2-inch thickness.

Melt butter in a saucepan over medium heat. Add mushrooms and cook until softened, about 4 minutes. Add garlic and thyme and cook until mushrooms are tender and most of the liquid has evaporated 4 to 5 minutes. Reduce heat to medium-low. Stir in cream cheese and season with salt. Cook and stir until cream cheese has completely melted. Remove from heat.

Spoon mushroom-cream mixture onto the chicken breasts—wrap chicken around the mixture and secure with toothpicks. Set chicken bundles, seam-side up, in a baking dish.

Bake in the preheated oven for 20 minutes. Remove from oven and brush with Dijon mustard. Sprinkle with Parmesan cheese and return to the oven.

Continue baking until no longer pink in the center, and the juices run clear, 15 to 20 minutes more. An instant-read thermometer inserted into the center should read at least 165 degrees F (74 degrees C). Discard toothpicks before serving.

Meat recipes

33) <u>**Steak N Gravy**</u>

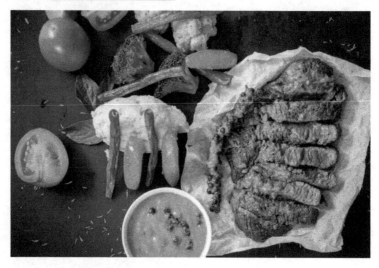

Ingredients

4 (4 ounces) venison steaks

1 cup all-purpose flour

2 tablespoons ground bay leaves

1 pinch salt and pepper

4 tablespoons olive oil, divided

1/2 onion, chopped

6 fresh mushrooms, sliced

1 tablespoon minced garlic

1 (10.5 ounces) can beef gravy

1/4 cup milk

Directions

Cut all fat and gristle off the meat, and pound each steak out with a meat tenderizer until they are thin but not tearing. In a shallow bowl, combine flour, bay leaf, salt, and pepper. Dredge steaks in the flour mixture until evenly coated.

Heat 1 tablespoon olive oil in a large, heavy skillet over medium heat. Saute onions until soft and translucent. Stir in mushrooms and garlic, and cook until tender. Remove from skillet and set aside. Heat remaining oil and fry each steak for 2 minutes on each side, or until golden brown. Return onion mixture to skillet. Stir in gravy and milk. Reduce heat, cover, and simmer for 30 to 40 minutes. Stir occasionally to prevent sticking.

34)   <u>Korean Ground Beef Bowl</u>

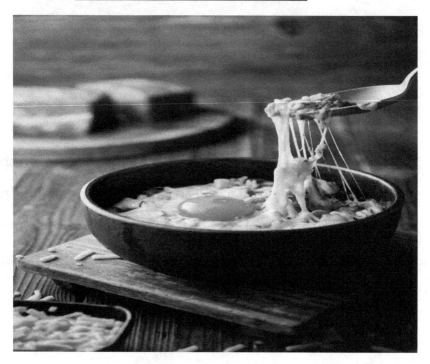

Ingredients

1 pound lean ground beef

5 cloves garlic, crushed

1 tablespoon freshly grated ginger

2 teaspoons toasted sesame oil

½ cup reduced-sodium soy sauce

⅓ cup light brown sugar

¼ teaspoon crushed red pepper

6 green onions, chopped, divided

4 cups hot cooked brown rice

1 tablespoon toasted sesame seeds

Directions

Heat a large skillet over medium-high heat. Add beef and cook, stirring and crumbling into small pieces until browned, 5 to 7 minutes. Drain excess grease.

Add garlic, ginger, and sesame oil, stirring until fragrant, about 2 minutes. Stir in soy sauce, brown sugar, and red pepper. Cook until some of the sauce absorbs into the beef, about 7 minutes. Add 1/2 of the chopped green onions.

Serve beef over hot cooked rice; garnished with sesame seeds and remaining green onions.

35) <u>Spinach Salad with Chicken, Avocado, and Goat Cheese</u>

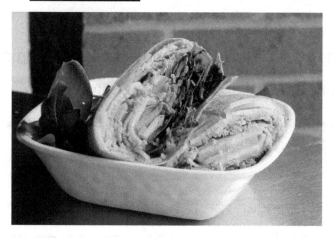

Ingredients

¼ cup pine nuts

8 cups chopped spinach

1 cup halved cherry tomatoes

1 ½ cups chopped cooked chicken

1 large avocado - peeled, pitted, and sliced

½ cup corn kernels

⅓ cup crumbled goat cheese

3 tablespoons white wine vinegar

2 tablespoons extra-virgin olive oil

1 tablespoon Dijon mustard

1 pinch salt and ground black pepper to taste

Directions

Heat a small skillet over medium-high heat—toast pine nuts in the hot skillet until lightly browned and fragrant, 3 to 5 minutes.

Put the spinach into a large salad bowl; top with pine nuts, tomatoes, chicken, avocado, corn kernels, and goat cheese.

Meat recipes

Beat white wine vinegar, olive oil, and Dijon mustard together in a small bowl until smooth; season with salt and pepper. Drizzle dressing over the salad and toss lightly to coat.

36) <u>**Bread Tacos**</u>

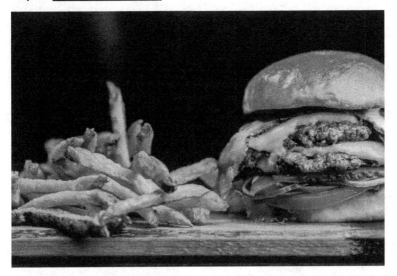

Ingredients

1 (15.5 ounces) can pinto beans, with liquid

½ cup Picante sauce, divided

1 pound ground beef

1 (1.25 ounce) package taco seasoning mix

Fry Bread:

2 cups all-purpose flour, or more as needed

1 tablespoon baking powder

1 teaspoon salt

1 cup milk

oil for frying

2 cups shredded iceberg lettuce

1 cup shredded Cheddar cheese

Directions

Combine beans and 2 tablespoons of Picante sauce in a small saucepan over low heat. Cook until heated through, about 5 minutes.

Combine ground beef and taco seasoning mix in a large skillet over medium-high heat; cook until browned, 5 to 8 minutes. Cover, and keep warm while you prepare the fry bread.

In a medium bowl, stir together the flour, baking powder, and salt. Stir in milk and mix until the dough comes together. Add more flour if necessary to be able to handle the dough.

On a floured surface, knead the dough until smooth, at least 5 minutes. Let the dough rest for 5 minutes. Break off 3/4 cup sized pieces of dough and shape into round discs 1/4 inch in thickness, making a thinner depressed area in the center.

Heat 1 1/2 inches oil in a large, deep heavy skillet to 365 degrees F (180 degrees C). Fry dough in the hot oil until golden on both sides, about 3 minutes per side. Drain on paper towels.

Top fry bread with beans, ground beef, lettuce, and Cheddar cheese. Spoon Picante sauce on top.

37) <u>Bacon</u>

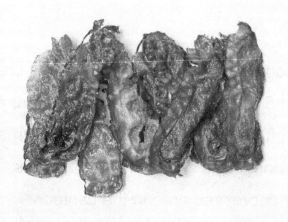

Ingredients

1/2 tablespoon butter

2 tablespoons chopped onion

3 slices stale bread, cut into cubes

1/4 cup shredded sharp Cheddar cheese

1 egg, beaten

1/4 teaspoon salt

1/4 teaspoon garlic powder

1/4 teaspoon ground black pepper

8 slices bacon

toothpicks

1 tablespoon bacon drippings

Directions

Melt butter in a skillet over medium-low heat and cook onion until soft and translucent, about 5 minutes.

Transfer to a bowl and add bread cubes, Cheddar cheese, egg, salt, garlic powder, and black pepper. Roll mixture into 8 equal-sized balls and wrap each ball in a slice of bacon. Use toothpicks to hold bacon in place.

Wipe the skillet clean. Melt bacon drippings over medium heat. Fry bacon balls in the skillet, constantly rolling until crisp, 15 to 18 minutes.

Notes:

_____

_____

_____

_____

_____

_____

Meat recipes

_____

_____

_____

_____

_____

_____